How To Seduce A Man

Find His Hot Buttons and Drive Him Crazy!

By Eugene Marks

I want to thank you for reading this book. You have read this book because you obviously have a problem. You need to seduce your man. Well, you came to the right place because I am a man and I know exactly what it takes to seduce a man because I am one.

So in this book we're going to cover some very important concepts that I think you're going to find extremely useful. One of the best things that I've learned has been, of course, from my own experience. But you obviously have your own experiences to base your own results from.

This book is going to provide you with sound techniques that I guarantee will seduce your man. If your man is not seduced by the information covered here, then you must not be applying it correctly.

If this doesn't work, your man is gay and seducing him would be impossible anyway, unless you're a gay man also.

You see, I know this works. This information has been shown to work time after time, over and over again.

It's probably not as difficult as you think. Here's the thing; if you're a woman you need to understand that you think in a completely different way than men do when it comes to seduction.

From this point forward keep in mind that I will be speaking in a general sense. Everyone is different and we all have different approaches to seduction. A man can be more like a woman sometimes, while a woman can be more like a man usually is. Everyone is different.

What I mean by this is that we all have the opportunity to step out of our old patterns of behavior and choose new ones. However I will be referring to women and men in the way history has generally shown their behavior to be like. I know there are exceptions to the rules.

How Women And Men Think Differently

It's been shown with women that one of the best ways to seduce a woman is a sense of humor. It allows a woman to feel more comfortable, more relaxed, and feel good when they are around this man.

So, for men, how do you do it?

What's the trick?

How do men tick?

How do they work?

What do they think about all of the time?

Well, it's been shown that men think about sex a lot. So seducing a man shouldn't be very difficult right?

Well, after you read this book I think you're going to find that what I'm going to show you will make it extremely simple, easy, practical, and you'll be seducing your man before you know it.

Here's the thing with women. Women find that what is familiar, safe, and comfortable, is often what allows them to open up, relax more. It puts them more in the mood.

With men, what they are more interested in is danger, excitement, the unknown. They want to feel adventurous like they're on the edge of their seat. The want to feel like what is coming to them is something that is unfamiliar to them, unknown, and they can't wait for the new adventure.

They're so excited. They're gleeful with anticipation of what is about to come. No pun intended.

So men enjoy mystery just like a woman does. But comfort bores men. Men tend to fantasize more than women. And men tend to look at sex as a destination.

Women look at sex as an enjoyable experience and tend to enjoy the entire experience. Women enjoy the kissing, the touching, the foreplay, the undressing, the slow touch, the feeling of skin against skin, and all of the senses involved.

Men enjoy this as well, but men tend to focus on wanting to get somewhere, rather than enjoying the moment.

Women have an incredible ability to be nurturing and soft in their experience; men tend to be harder and less present in sex.

Now, of course, I don't know your man. Every man is different. But, as a general rule, men tend to enjoy sex for the sake of the experience but also because of the feeling of power that it gives them.

This feeling of power appeals to the ego of the man. Men and women each have an ego but the man's ego tends to be stroked by the feeling of accomplishment.

This is why sex is looked upon as a conquest from a man. A man will feel proud of himself for getting a job done or being seen by their partner as powerful and influential.

They believe that if they score with the hot chick, this means something about them. If a man gives his woman an orgasm, this means something about him and how influential he must be.

There are some men who are willing to give up the ego and enjoy sex more for the experience of sex, rather the sense of accomplishment.

But, some men relate to sex as a way of making them feel more powerful. Having sex can make them feel important; it can make men feel like they are somebody special.

But men also have higher testosterone levels then women. So there is a more primal urge in existence with men than with women for the need and desire for sex.

It can be so overwhelming and so thought consuming to a man, that he is not able to think straight at times. When he is in the mood, his brain is consumed with hormones such as dopamine and adrenaline and he is not consciously aware of it. He just must have sex, and he wants it NOW.

This is the level that you need to relate to a man. You want to relate to his primal urges because this is the way to seduce a man in to wanting to have sex with you.

In my other book, "How To Seduce Women", I take a completely different approach. Men and women are truly polar opposites when it comes to seduction so the techniques with the exception of a few, are completely different.

Appeal to a man's hormones, not to his logical brain. As you will soon see, we will talk about the five senses, and how to use those five senses in order to appeal to his lustful brain.

The 5 Senses

Now, of course, we all know about the five senses. We see. We touch. We smell. We hear and we taste. The biggest senses that will trigger a man's sex drive will be touch, what he smells, what he sees, and what he hears.

Touch

Touch can be very, very exciting. I can remember a moment back in high school when a girl I knew approached me. She stood right in front of me and gently touched my hand. I don't recall what she was talking to me about. All I remember was suddenly I felt extremely excited inside.

I felt my whole body go crazy right down to my very tippy toes all the way to my fingertips, all the way up to my head. In fact, my blood started to rush to my head and I started to blush.

I remember that very well. So it's amazing how **touch** can have a tremendous effect on seducing a man. Suddenly I felt important in someone else's eyes. I felt desired which was incredibly powerful and almost overwhelming. It was addictive in fact.

So that's one thing that you can do is touch. Because, if you're not used to touching your man and this is a newer relationship, just a simple hand stroke or light rub on the back can make a man go crazy.

Now, if your relationship is more grounded, and you've been in a relationship for a while, and you're looking for the right way to touch a man, I do recommend massages.

Now, there are a couple of different ways to massage. You can do gentle, and light, or hard and rough. And either way you're going to find that if you go to extremes on either type of massage you're going to find this helpful in relaxing a man.

Yes, men enjoy massages as well as women. It makes them feel cared for. It makes them feel proud to be a man. And when they get touched by a woman it makes them feel good.

A massage can also be an opportunity to role play which we will discuss later. How many stories have you heard of massages giving a man an erection?

A massage can relax a man and alter his state of mind. If he has been tense about something, by massaging his shoulders, you can change his state of mind and give him an opportunity to get in touch with his body, instead of his mind.

As I mentioned earlier, seducing a man really isn't that difficult. I think what most women probably want; is to figure out a way to keep their man interested and keep him excited.

Sight

Really what it's about my good lady is you have feminine features that are really attractive to men. So you'll want to highlight your attractive physical features, but not give away too much. You want to tease his eyes.

By teasing a man's eyes, he can now let his imagination take over and begin to fantasize about what those features look like without clothing.

For example, if you were to show up to the workplace completely naked you would be giving away too much too soon. You want to show a little bit of skin. Be classy about it, but not show too much.

So what are the two most attractive features that men often think about? Breasts and the buttocks. The breasts and the buttocks are some of the best qualities and features you can show off.

How often have you heard the question, "Are you a breast man or an ass man?"

Look at your body and decide what your best features are. You know your own body best but you can certainly ask your friends in order to get other opinions.

Maybe there are features you can show off that you think are extremely attractive. Maybe you have an extremely attractive wrist that you can show off. I'm sort of kidding but my point is that you want to make yourself look as attractive as possible.

Seriously though, breasts, buttocks, and stomach are probably the three best areas that you can show off in order to attract a man. By the way I don't mean the inside organ of your stomach. I mean the belly.

As I mentioned earlier, men are extremely visually interested, and what they see visually, allows an idea to be planted in their mind of the idea of sex. I'll talk more on this later.

And what you want to do is allow him to plant the idea in hYou can't force it upon him. Men have to come up with the idea on their own. As I mentioned earlier, touch is really important.

So if you can find a way to just gently touch your man and tease a little bit with touch, along with dressing your best for visual appeal; you're going to find this will often drive your man crazy.

Sounds

The other important topic I want to talk about when I mention the five senses is sound.

So there are sounds that you can make that will simulate sex. Sexy sounds can plant the idea in a man's mind of the **idea** of sex.

For example, if you moan, you can use a slightly more high pitched voice. You can also use a slightly more innocent type voice, or you can show your man that you are a little bit vulnerable.

Just by changing your voice to be more seductive like this will help improve your chances of seducing him and making him do what you want.

So in your voice, you want to use higher tones. You also want to use lower tones. You want to fluctuate your tones a little bit. You'll want to moan a little, because any sound that might simulate sex will have him associate your voice with sounds that stimulate his mind and body for sex.

Even your heavy breathing can plant the idea in the man's mind of sex because there is heavy breathing in sex and foreplay. Play around with this idea and be subtle about it. Don't overdo it.

Smell

Of course, one of the best things that I like on my lady is nice perfume. A little touch of perfume on the collar bone can help plant the idea in a man's mind of wanting to explore.

This primal urge of wanting to explore, based on what we smell, comes from back in the cavemen days.

A long time ago, when we smelled a piece of meat out there in the woods somewhere, it drove us to a point of curiosity and lust, and attracted us to it.

Well, this primal sense is no different with perfume. Only this time instead of the smell of food he's lusting for, you are now the piece of meat he wants to devour.

I'm not saying that you season yourself with garlic salt and barbecue sauce. A nice smelling perfume can do wonders for seducing your man.

Taste

Taste can be just as important, but rarely do you hear of seducing a man with a good tasting bunt cake. In general; if there is a pleasant taste in our mouth it can recall memories of other times when a similar food was being consumed.

So this means you can train your man like Pavlov's dog to lust for you because of a taste based earlier memory.

If you are not familiar with Pavlov's dog, Pavlov was a scientist who was able to train his dog and let his dog know that dinner was ready by ringing a bell.

He noticed that the bell ringing would trigger the dog to drool because the dog was excited about the food that was thought by the dog to soon be arriving in his bowl.

So imagine if you combined the other senses; such as hearing your sexy moans while he is eating whip cream on a pie. Then, later in the bedroom he is licking whip cream off your nipples and you are using the same moaning sounds.

Do you see how you can train his mind to anticipate sex by triggering memories of taste and his other senses at the same time?

Experiment with certain foods and tastes. Also, you can use food to increase his sex drive. An example of aphrodisiacs include asparagus, bananas, chocolate, figs, and oysters.

Unattainable

As I mentioned earlier, women tend to be attracted to what's familiar, safe, and known, which is often why they like a sense of humor. It makes them feel good and comfortable.

Men, on the other hand, tend to be attracted to what they feel is perhaps separate or distant from them. In other words, men can often feel attracted to what they believe they can't have.

So try to think of yourself as a goddess, something that's untouchable, that cannot be possessed, very difficult to obtain, a rare gem perhaps.

By thinking of yourself in this way, you're going to find that this is going to be a quality that will make a man very excited and very interested in you.

He'll see you as a challenge. He'll see you as something that he needs to strive for in order to obtain.

So, if you look at yourself and see yourself as something that is an object that cannot be obtained, that is difficult to get, and that you are a rare gem, you will soon become a hunted object by your man.

This dates back to high school. In fact, in high school, teenage boys often desired that girl in high school who was popular, who was surrounded by friends, and who just seemed like the kind of person who was unobtainable for them.

This unconscious behavior drove the teenage boys crazy. Which brings me to another important point.

Self Image

Your self-image is going to be an important aspect to seducing your man. You need to actually see yourself as the person you want to become. So I actually invite you now to take a few moments.

Take a few deep breaths. Take five minutes of a good silent deep breath right now. Allow your body to relax.

Try your best to empty your mind of thought. After you have done this, grab a piece of paper and start writing down exactly what this dream person looks like.

What does she smell like?

Who does she associate with?

What kind of body does she have?

Be as detailed as possible.

When you can start to see yourself as this beautiful seductive woman, you're going to have a better shot of seducing your man rather then if you thought of yourself as some shlumpie housewife or just a worn out and tired mom, who wears expandable sweat pants all the time.

Instead; see yourself as an erotic sexual object and you will be amazed by how much of a difference this will make in your seducing a man.

Why He Doesn't Want Sex

Now, I know that not every case is exactly the same, but sometimes your man may not want to have sex. Now, here are some reasons why your man may not want to have sex.

So if you're a woman in a sexless relationship or marriage, and you're not sure why; we will now cover the possible causes. You may be trying to figure out why your man does not want sex.

I mean, after all, aren't men supposed to have this insatiable sex appetite, and want it all the time? You know the stereotype I speak of.

Well, why would a man refuse to be sexually intimate with his wife or girlfriend, especially when the wife or girlfriend is doing everything she can think of to spark the desire inside him?

Even though we've all grown up with the idea that men are lustful, sex hungry animals, you know, that necessarily isn't exactly always the case.

There are a lot of factors that can affect whether or not the man is sexually hungry or not. There can be numerous factors.

In fact, some reasons can range from work stress, just being tired, side effects of medications, but, sometimes those are deterrents.

A man who has a close and loving relationship with his wife or girlfriend will still be intimate and physically affectionate with her, even if sexual intercourse is a problem.

The fact is that the main reason why men don't want to have sex with their wife is because something has come between the man and woman in their relationship. This is something that a lot of people don't necessarily expect.

So, yes, men are interested physically in sex, but physical attraction is not just what they're interested in. There is always the emotional aspect that you can't always see.

A lot of men have graduated from that teenage horny stage; where they want to have sex with just anything. Now that they have grown up and they need to feel strong emotional connection in order to be interested in sex.

If you're having trouble seducing your man and you feel like things are fine physically, then, there might be some emotional issues that you may not be aware of.

This is often a subject that is not talked about, but is important to be addressed.

Business Meetings

One of the best things that my wife and I do is sit down together and have a weekly business meeting. And in the weekly business meeting we have an opportunity to address any issues that are in our relationship.

Now these issues may not seem like they're directly related to the sex life, but in actuality, they are.

Because when you can clear the air with your partner, you can start to feel free to be yourself, and feel free around the other person, as well as feel like you can desire the other person sexually without reservation.

In a relationship, the partners stop seeing each other like they did when the relationship was new and fresh. Each partner isn't necessarily seeing the other person. Instead they're seeing all of the stress, worry, resentment, or topics they need to talk about with that person.

So in our business meeting the first thing that we we talk about is taking the time to acknowledge and appreciate each other. We both get a chance to share what we appreciate about each other at the beginning of our business meeting.

This is an important first step because we all need to be acknowledged and appreciated. It's shown that employees will often work for less money at a workplace they feel appreciation at, then a workplace where there is more money but no appreciation.

Telling someone how much you appreciate them is extremely attractive. This must be done without strings attached or expectation of reciprocation. Otherwise it's not true appreciation.

The next thing that we do is address any future plans that are coming up; things that we need to talk about that are coming up in the future, such as events, or our kid's school activities, our day trips or fieldtrips we will be taking soon.

Then, we talk about weeds. **Weeds** are anything that you might be holding resentment about in the relationship. There's a certain way that we actually share these weeds. As you can imagine sharing issues you have with your partner can be tricky so you want to share in such a way that the relationship becomes stronger.

We actually made a special card that we pass back and forth to each other and whoever has the card gets to talk. The other person who has the card does not get to talk. They only get to listen.

Once that person is done sharing their weed, the other person will recite back to the other partner what it was he or she just said.

This allows the partner to feel like they've been heard. And when someone feels like they've been heard it creates disappearance and the issues are easier to get resolved in a relationship that way.

The weeds may take some time to get resolved because after all, a real relationship will have problems. But if each partner can promise to be patient and to listen to the other partner, this exercise can do wonders for a relationship.

So once those types of issues get resolved, intimacy can come back into the relationship and it becomes easier to seduce, or engage in some kind of other sexual activity, or any type of activity for that matter.

After sharing our weeds and getting our issues resolved, one partner will listen while the other partner reads a dream statement. The dream statement is simply a statement that you and your partner can create about your relationship.

The dream statement is not about what your relationship looked like, but rather what your relationship will be. It is your dream relationship.

Our dream statement says that our relationship will be passionate, joyous, open, and fun.

If you are in a relationship I suggest you have a weekly business meeting so that you can clear the air, and talk about any issues which may make it difficult to have the kind of relationship you want.

Role play

A man's imagination will be the most powerful tool to seducing him. A man's imagination makes him obsess about an idea that has been planted in his mind.

If he has an idea of something he wants, he will tear down walls to satisfy his primal urge and conquer the idea he has planted in his mind.

This is why **role playing** can be so powerful to seducing men. A man gets to use his imagination and fulfill on one of his fantasies.

If you have costumes and you can find new unfamiliar physical places to act out and **role play**, this will make sex more exciting to him because he will get to completely abandon his old patterns of thinking and access new parts of his brain.

It will feel dangerous and adventurous. As we've discussed earlier; this unknown territory can get a man excited.

Examples of role playing could be:

The massage therapist who seduces him into sex

Meeting a "stranger" at the local bar

The delivery man who delivers more than just one package

An "affair" with another sex partner

Two co-workers having sex at the office

Two actors rehearsing a sex scene

You get the point. You could go on and on with these **role playing** scenarios. I'm sure you could come up with some good ones yourself. If you enjoy them, you will probably put more creative energy into them. So be sure it is a scenario you enjoy also.

Conclusion

I hope that this book was useful to you. I want to thank you for reading it. Thank you so much. I look forward to hearing about how this has helped you have a more enriching and fulfilling relationship with a man.

Or if your aim is seduction without a relationship I trust you found the ideas in here helpful and very valuable to you also

Remember we get out of things what we put in. If you want to seduce him beyond your wildest dreams, I strongly urge you to take the principles covered in this book and apply them immediately.

You may not be perfect at first. But the more energy and attention you give these concepts, the more you will get back. It is like an investment. At first you may not see immediate results, however with time, action, and persistent faith you will see results beyond your dreams.

How To Sext Your Way Into His Pants

By Eugene Marks

Introduction

Thank you for picking up a copy of this book. I know this is an exciting and interesting topic and yet the idea of sexting is relatively new in our society. It used to be, we didn't have this kind of technology and now we do.

Sexting is not just limited to texting, and it's not just limited to the cell phone. You can sext through video, audio, voice mail, images, and messages. You can also communicate through email, not just text messages.

What we are going to show you in this book is not only how you can use this technology to seduce men and have the desired sexual outcome that you are looking for; we are also going to show you a little bit of the dangers of this as well, so you can avoid some of the pitfalls that people have made when it comes to sexting.

I'm going to give you some real examples but the intention is not that you follow exactly what I suggest. Instead I'm giving you an idea and what you should do is take that idea and run with it.

I'm being pretty vague in this book intentionally. This is your creative plan, and I don't want you to do the exact plan I lay out. Instead I want you to think outside the box and use your own methods.

Mostly the information inside this book is best for women who want to sext a man crazy! As you'll soon see, this can work really well, and it can be fun too.

The Art of Sexting

The actual art of sexting is very simple. It only requires a few methods and a few techniques. I am sure if you use your imagination and think outside the box, you can find creative ways to seduce a man through sexting.

But what I want to talk to you about is laying the foundation for good sexting. And the way we do that is that we talk about the mindset of a man and we also talk about creating your desired outcome.

See, I believe that by manifesting through our own mind power, we can create the desired outcome of what we are looking for. For example, if we want to seduce a man, then we are going to want to think about how **exactly** this is going to look.

We must have a picture in our mind in order to help us manifest our thoughts into reality. I want you to stop what you are doing right now, and I want you to grab a blank sheet of paper, or I want you to get on your computer and create a new word document. Now begin to right down your own vision; a clear idea of what you want this experience to look like. How do you want this to go?

This is an exercise that I teach in a lot of my books and the reason I do this is that if people can get a clear idea of what it is exactly that they want, then they can have it a lot quicker, and faster, and easier. Most people don't get what they want, because they are not clear about exactly what is it that they want.

So go ahead and begin to write down ideas, thoughts and fantasies about how this is going to look. How are you going to seduce him? How do you *want* to seduce him? What is it that you want to have happen as a result of your sext messaging?

Don't just jump into sext messaging. Be clear about the dangers and the risks, like we will talk about later, and be clear about what you want to have happen as well.

Once you have done this, you can start to create your plan out clearly. And I bet you'll come up with some pretty creative ideas on how you can make him excited and aroused. It's really not that difficult to arouse a man. It starts with your mind; this is the creative tool to bringing you and him more pleasure.

Let's face it, men think about sex all the time. So what we are going to talk about is how a man thinks and how it's different from women. In this way, you can tap into that part of the man's brain that will be stimulated by your sexting, before you begin doing your sext messaging, images or video.

First off, you have to understand how a man thinks. A man fantasizes about sex. He desires it. He particularly desires what it is he cannot have.

Not only is it important that you create the outcome that you want, and you believe and it is clear to you how your sexting will go, it is also important that you see yourself as a sexual goddess.

You must be confident in how you portray yourself. Since you are confident, you can take your sexting to a new level by creating a story. Keep it interesting and keep a saga going.

Sexting once is exciting, but creating a whole story and a fantasy for him, will make it even more exciting for him. Keep this in mind. The way a man is different than a woman is that a man has more testosterone, which means he does not think about sex logically. He can't.

The testosterone in his body has caused him to *react* to what he perceives through his senses, and that's the way a man thinks when it comes to sex. He's not really thinking.

He's just **reacting** to what is going on around him. You want to tap into the primal part of his brain. He just wants sex. Nobody says they want sex a week from now or months from now. The part of the brain that thinks ahead is not the same part where men think about sex. When people want sex, they want it NOW, and that's the kind of urgency that you want to tap into in his brain with what you show him in your sexting.

If you've ever watched porn, you can see why men love it. The women make sounds of pleasure. These sounds of pleasure trigger a man's brain. If you are doing videos or even audio messages, be sure to moan and breathe heavy like women do in porn.

Also you can see in porn, how much a woman's ass is shown on camera in the bending over position. One of men's favorite sexual positions is doggy style. If you can bend over and show photos, it will trigger his mind into hyper activity. He'll wish he could stick his dick in you so bad, he can taste it.

Dangers

Before we go any further, let's talk about the pitfalls, and some of the dangers of sexting. I have heard horrible stories. What can happen in sexting, is sometimes people will produce content, images, videos, texts and send it to their partner, and then later, their partner will break up with them or not have made a real commitment to the relationship.

And then that partner will release the information that you just sexted them, into the digital world; it may be on Facebook or their blog, even YouTube. So you have to be extremely careful when you do this kind of activity. You don't want this to information to come across the wrong way and released into the wrong hands.

I always recommend with sexting, that you do this with somebody you trust and you love, and you have been in a committed relationship with this person for a long time, because if you are not cautious; you might end up having your images or your videos all over the internet. Nobody wants that. It can be a very painful and embarrassing experience for someone.

In July 2010, an 18 year old high school student committed suicide after a nude photo she had transmitted via her cell phone to her boyfriend, was also sent to 100s of teenagers in her school. Students who saw the photo allegedly harassed her.

It's unusual that kids are being arrested for child pornography, but sexting under the age of 18 is against the law. Breaking the law is another thing you never want to do. It can be embarrassing to say the least. Currently laws are being made against sexting because it is considered Child Pornography. So, be careful!!

I not only recommend that you wait until you are at least 18, I recommend that you do this with a committed partner and that you wait to do this with someone you truly trust and love.

The damage that can happen from sexting, can take a huge emotional toll. I think you understand by now from the example I talked about with the girl who committed suicide, just how serious and dangerous it can be.

It's ok if sexting is not for you. It's not for everyone. Just because your friends are doing it, doesn't mean you have to do it either. You are perfect just the way you are. Don't sext someone if your self esteem depends on how another person will react to you. There are plenty of other ways to seduce a man.

I also recommend that you make it clear with your partner what time of day you will sext. This way they don't ask someone to check their phone to see who just texted them while they step away. Ask your partner to clear their phone of any images or videos immediately after you sent them.

How To Sext With Video

I want to talk about the exciting parts of sexting and how it can be beneficial to you in your relationship and create more exciting sex for you and your partner. Because that's what it is all about. I don't want to focus too much on the negative because I have already talked about the negative.

Now, let's talk about the positives. Sexting can be done from just your phone, but it can also be done via email, and it doesn't necessarily have to be in the form of text. It can be in the form of picture and it can be in the form of video.

Let's talk about video, because video can be one of the most pleasing ways to engage your partner in a way that you never would have thought was possible before. Imagine sending your partner a video and showing vulnerable parts of your body and pleasing yourself.

This can really create arousal in your partner. Now, if you are doing this, you can sort of tease your partner a little bit. You don't have to show the whole thing (by this I mean your entire body, privates and all). You don't even have to show vulnerable body parts right away. You can do your video sexting in a short series. I'm talking about short videos that only last a few minutes.

You can start off for example, by just showing the belly. Then quickly show the face, and then you can start to pull down your shirt just a little bit, and then cut the video. But before you cut the video, let them know that the video that they *really* want to see, will be the next video.

By doing this, you can create a teasing effect, and make your partner want more and more. Then, on your next video, you can show a little bit more. You can start to peel your underwear down a little bit and then you can start to take off your bra. Then, you can start to reach your hands down your pants and touch your vagina. Right after you touch your vagina, cut the video. (At this point, all he can see is that you've reached your hand down your underwear.)

Then, on the next video, that's when you can just let it all go and show everything, or you could still hold back in order to make him think about the video he just saw, all day long.

The next video could leave right where the last video ended. Only this time you masturbate, almost to climax. Right before climax, you cut the video.

That's one possible way you can seduce a man with video.

Caution: if you are using video content and say for example you are using video hosting, such as YouTube, you want to use the Private settings. Don't use the Unlisted and don't use the Public settings. The Public settings will allow everybody to see it and you want to have special security access that only he can see in order to see the video content that you are looking for. Make sure you know how to take a video down if you need to, and that you are the only person with access into your video hosting account.

Text Your Way To Better Sex

Now, let's talk about how you can do it with writing text. Writing text can be very powerful as well; many times it can be safer than video or pictures also. You can say messages like, "I am horny" or "I want you" or "Where are you I need your lovin right now".

These are all samples of messages you can use in sexting. You have to use your own language and find what works for you.

But the one thing that you want to watch out for with writing messages is; you don't know who has control of the other person's phone, and it's the same thing with video or with your pictures. You don't know who really has control of the other phone. So you want to be careful with what you say, and what you show, because you never know who could see your message.

Also, you don't know who could have access to your partner's email account. Make sure your messages, images or videos will be sent to an email of someone you trust completely.

I have heard horror stories of people's in laws getting the messages from their partner's phone, instead of the person who it was intended for. So watch out!

You can always create a secret code with your lover. For example: **IWYB** could mean: **I Want You Badly**. That's just an example. Use your own wording that works for you and your partner.

Sexy Photos

Let's talk about pictures. Pictures can be extremely exciting as well. And just like with your video, you don't have to show everything right away. You can tease a little bit. You can show just the belly or a photo that shows that you are just starting to peel off your underwear, but you haven't stripped enough to reveal any privates.

Then you can take a photo of your hand reaching down your pants. Then, of course you can always show the whole thing. You can spread your legs and show the whole vagina.

If you need help on ideas for sexy photos to send for sexting, you can do research online and search porno websites. You can also buy a copy of Playboy, Hustler magazines, etc.

I know that pornographic images can be disturbing and completely fake. But the point is that you get ideas on how to pose and show off your body, in a way that will arouse your partner. Think of it as research and don't compare yourself to the actresses with low self esteem. You don't have to sext him a photo of you doing a gang bang, just because those women are doing it. In fact, that's just sound advice; don't do a gangbang just because everyone else is doing it.

There are certain parts of the body that are extremely attractive to men. The breast, the buttocks, and the vagina, are all parts of your body you can show to get a man in the mood. These are the parts of the body that really arouse men.

So, of course, you can show off these parts to create arousal in your partner. With photos, text and video, you can tease your partner by letting him know that you are going to be at a certain location; and by letting him know that you are going to be at a certain location, you can take control of the whole conversation that way, if you want to.

You can let him know that you are not going to text any more. If he wants to see you in person, he can meet you at XXX location at XXX time. You can even text a photo of yourself at that location in a sexy t-shirt.

The Advantages of Sexting

What do you suppose might be some of the advantages of sexting, versus actually meeting someone face to face? Why are we so attracted to the digital form of entertainment? Men love to use their imagination. A man's imagination is extremely powerful in triggering his desire for sex.

Men love to use their imagination and through messages, through pics and through videos, men get to use their imagination in ways they never would have done before if they were with you physically. They get to *fantasize*.

Imagine you are touching yourself with your hand in your video or picture, and they get to imagine that it's their hand that's touching you instead of yours.

Another aspect of text messaging and digital content that cannot be done through the physical way, is the idea of **not** being able to have something. It's been shown that men really desire what it is that they cannot have. Imagine if there's a video of you doing a naked dance but he can't be with you right now.

This will drive him nuts, because he cannot actually be there with you and if you use this in the right way, it can be a very powerful way to turn him on and make him really desire you. He'll be thinking about that sext message and recalling the memory over and over. He will stew upon the idea, letting it boil and fester inside him.

You can use this as a seduction technique. If you've been having trouble seducing this guy, then maybe texting or sexting is the way to go for you.

Conclusion

You'll notice that this is a very short book and there's a reason for that – **because you don't need a lot of information**. I can certainly overload you with ideas and information. But you don't need them. Really what you want to do is practice the information that has been shown here. Once you've practiced this information, you will internalize it and know way more then any book can show you. We've shown the dangers and we've shown why we don't want to do this in an illegal way.

But we have also shown how you can use powerful content to seduce a man and why sexting is such an incredible form of arousal for a man. It allows them to use the fantasy part of their mind and imagine themselves in a situation where they are not physically already. The current pain and the desire for pleasure, make him obsess about being with you.

Human beings are motivated by two things; one is to avoid pain and the other is to bring them self closer to pleasure. Very few human beings actually like being where they exist in the moment right now. We are often reaching for more, or desire more, in order to avoid feeling our current feelings. Texting and digital content allows you and your partner to escape into a fantasy world.

So, I want you to go out there and have fun! Use this information and through experimentation you are going to become even better at sexting a man into the bedroom.

I hope that this book is both useful to you and that you use it for the power of good. I hope that you only use it to build your self-esteem and you don't have any detrimental effects from this.

It is my dream and my hope that you have the lifestyle that you desire. I know that you can have incredible sex by using the information here. But most importantly, I want you to take this information and develop your own methods.

You know in your own mind, how to sext correctly. Don't you? You know how to create this incredible arousal for a man and you are aware of the risks. It's just a matter of going out there and doing it.

Thank you so much for reading this book. You should definitely check out some of my other books, because my other books fill in the missing gaps for how to tap into a man's mind. I believe understanding the opposite sex will help you with your sexting as well. Thank you so much.

Disclaimer:

Thank You

Thank you for reading this book. It is a pleasure to provide quality content for readers like you. To read more great books by this author or publisher please review a list of our other books below. I hope you found this book helpful.

Do you have positive comments?

Your Amazon reviews help other readers in selecting quality books like this one. Please take a moment and review this book now while the information is fresh in your mind.

In addition to providing quality eBooks, we also provide quality training and systems to those wanting to make money online. You can connect with the publisher, Mat Gunnufson on facebook at www.facebook.com/mat.gunnufson to learn more. You may visit Mat's website at www.prosperwithmc.com and watch a free video and begin making money immediately upon joining.

Current Books Published by Mat Gunnufson.

Look For These Books On Amazon Kindle Today!

Muscle Strength-Granny To Manly by Mat Gunnufson

Make Money From Internet Marketing by Mat Gunnufson

Photo Business-How I Made Over 18000 Profit Per Month by Mat Gunnufson

Dating For Teens by Mat Gunnufson

How To Fall In Love by Mat Gunnufson

Stop Sex Addiction by Eugene Marks

Addiction Recovery by Eugene Marks

How To Seduce Women by Eugene Marks

How To Seduce A Man by Eugene Marks

How To End An Affair by Eugene Marks

Self Esteem For Kids by Mary Graham

End Depression by Mary Graham

Get People To Like You by Mary Graham

Dealing With Jealousy by Mary Graham

Work Addiction by Mary Graham

www.ingramcontent.com/pod-product-compliance
Lightning Source LLC
Chambersburg PA
CBHW070131290526
45789CB00005B/2204